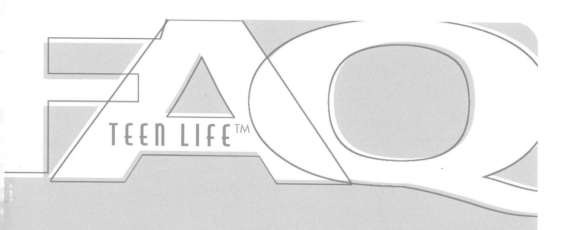

TEEN LIFE™

FREQUENTLY ASKED QUESTIONS ABOUT

Antidepressants

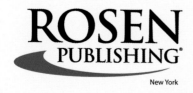

Judy
Monroe
Peterson

ROSEN
PUBLISHING®
New York

To my friend Lois

Published in 2010 by The Rosen Publishing Group, Inc.
29 East 21st Street, New York, NY 10010

Library of Congress Cataloging-in-Publication Data

Peterson, Judy Monroe.
Frequently asked questions about antidepressants / Judy Monroe Peterson.—1st ed.
    p. cm.—(FAQ: teen life)
Includes index.
ISBN 978-1-4358-3547-4 (library binding)
1. Antidepressants—Popular works. 2. Depression, Mental—Popular works. I. Title.
RM332.P48 2010
615'.78—dc22

2009018962

Manufactured in Malaysia

CPSIA Compliance Information: Batch #TWW10YA: For Further Information contact Rosen Publishing, New York, New York at 1-800-237-9932

Contents

one

WHAT ARE ANTIDEPRESSANTS?

Antidepressants are medications prescribed by doctors to treat depression and other disorders, such as panic and eating disorders and anxiety. Currently, more than twenty different antidepressants are available for adults and teens. Most can be taken as a capsule, tablet, or liquid. The U.S. Food and Drug Administration (FDA) regulates antidepressants and all other prescription medications.

Antidepressants are not stimulants. They do not make you feel overly excited, happy, or peppy. Antidepressants reduce the amount of excessive depression that you were feeling. They help you feel the way you did before you became depressed. Antidepressants are commonly used in the United States. In 2008, the Agency for Healthcare Research and Quality reported that people in the United States filled nearly 170 million prescriptions for antidepressants in

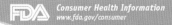

FDA Consumer Health Information
www.fda.gov/consumer

www.fda.gov/consumer/updates/antidepressants010909.html

Understanding Antidepressant Medications

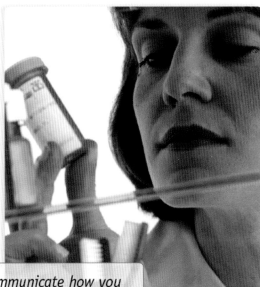

Depression affects about 121 million people worldwide and is a leading cause of disability, according to the World Health Organization (WHO).

"In my experience as a practicing psychiatrist, I've seen that many people with depression don't realize that they have the condition or that it's treatable," says Mitchell Mathis, M.D., deputy director of the Division of Psychiatry Products at the Food and Drug Administration (FDA).

Some who suffer from depression don't recognize the symptoms, or they attribute them to lack of sleep or a poor diet. Others realize they are depressed, but they feel too fatigued or ashamed to seek help.

Not all depression requires treatment with medication.

It's important to communicate how you are feeling so that your physician can evaluate the medication's effectiveness.

Photodisc

The Food and Drug Administration (FDA) is an agency of the U.S. Department of Health and Human Services and is responsible for regulating the safety of antidepressants and other drugs.

2005. The use of antidepressants among people ages ten to nineteen continues to increase.

Feeling Down

Being in a bad mood every now and then is normal and a part of everyday life. Most teens feel sad or down sometimes. Getting rejected, breaking up, or being turned down for a date are common reasons why teens feel sad or disappointed. Occasionally, you may feel blue or out-of-sorts for no particular reason at all, but you still participate in regular activities like going to school and spending time with friends. Your sadness or unhappy feelings are temporary. They usually pass in a day or in a few days.

Sometimes, a difficult event may occur that sends some people into a depression. If your parents get divorced, a beloved pet dies, or a close friend is in a horrible accident, you might feel shock, anger, or deep sadness. Over time, people usually work through their grief and adjust to the changes in their lives. However, if these feelings persist for an abnormally long time, you might have depression.

Depression

According to the National Institute of Mental Health, about 14.8 million adults in the United States have depression. Nearly two million teenagers (ages twelve to eighteen) are affected by this disorder as well. In April 2009, the U.S. Preventive Services Task Force, which sets guidelines for doctors on many health issues,

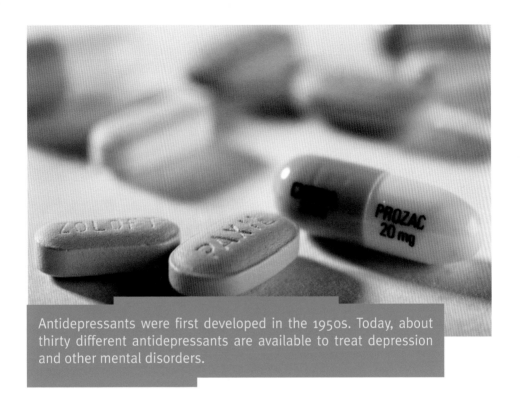

Antidepressants were first developed in the 1950s. Today, about thirty different antidepressants are available to treat depression and other mental disorders.

recommended that all American teenagers get screened for depression, as long as there are appropriate screening tests to ensure accurate diagnosis, treatment, and follow-up care. This serious medical illness affects emotions, thoughts, behaviors, and health. People might feel hopeless, deeply unhappy, or unconnected to friends and family members. They lose interest in relationships, school, and social activities.

Depression can continue for several weeks, months, or even longer. The symptoms vary for each person. Common symptoms include feeling negative, sleeping too much or too little, and weight gain or loss. Small tasks, such as making your bed or brushing your teeth, can seem like a huge undertaking. In very serious cases, people may even have thoughts of hurting themselves. Depression can usually be treated successfully, though, and a variety of treatments are available. Treatment for teens usually includes therapy or a combination of antidepressant medications and therapy.

How Antidepressants Work

Researchers are not exactly sure how antidepressants change the chemistry of the brain. Your brain is made up of billions of neurons that communicate with one another. Neurons pass messages to other neurons by releasing many different types of chemical substances called neurotransmitters. The main neurotransmitters that antidepressants affect are serotonin, norepinephrine, and, to a lesser extent, dopamine.

Neurotransmitters are released from storage in small "bubbles" called vesicles, which are located at the ends of neurons (nerve cells). These biochemicals cross the gaps between neurons, called synapses, and then bind to neurotransmitter receptors on nearby neurons. Messages that move from neuron to neuron can be about thoughts, emotions, behavior, body temperature, appetite, or other body functions. The types and amounts of neurotransmitters control how neurons communicate in the brain. When neurotransmitters finish their work, the sending neuron usually reabsorbs them in a process called reuptake. Then the neurotransmitters can be released again later.

Sometimes, the reuptake of serotonin or norepinephrine occurs too soon. As a result, the brain does not have enough of

This computer artwork shows the action of antidepressants called selective serotonin reuptake inhibitors (SSRIs). The SSRIs (pink) work at synapses to block the reuptake of serotonin (orange). More of the neurotransmitter serotonin is then available.

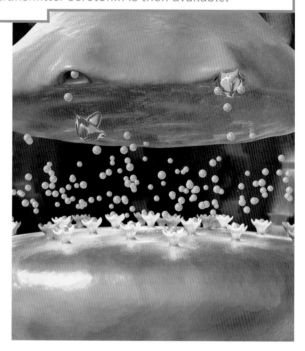

the neurotransmitter. This can cause depression. Each type of antidepressant works differently. Some antidepressants slow the reuptake process of serotonin or norepinephrine in the brain. Other antidepressants interact directly with the receptors that release these neurotransmitters. In all cases, antidepressants cause an increase in the levels of serotonin or norepinephrine that stick around in the synapses. This process allows more neurotransmitters to interact with their receptors, which generally improves people's moods.

The receptors take some time to adapt in different ways as the levels of neurotransmitters increase. It is not known if the number of receptors increases or the ability of neurotransmitters to bind to their receptors increases. Perhaps it is a combination of the two. Researchers think that the changes in the receptors cause mood to improve, but they do not completely understand yet how this happens. Receptors usually take from two to four weeks to adjust. This means it takes that long, or a little longer, for most antidepressants to take full effect in the body.

Possible Risk of Suicidal Behavior

When doctors prescribe an antidepressant for teens, their first choice is often a type of antidepressant called selective serotonin reuptake inhibitors (SSRIs). Most teens have few side effects when using SSRIs. If side effects occur, they usually disappear within a month. Compared to other types of antidepressants, SSRIs are less likely to be harmful if teens take an overdose. This is important because teens with depression are already at an increased risk for suicide.

Some people think that the use of antidepressants increases the risk of suicide in children and teens. The FDA has analyzed twenty-four past studies of about 4,400 teens and children who had taken antidepressants. No suicides had occurred in the studies. However, the agency stated that SSRIs may cause a very small proportion of teens to be at an increased risk of suicidal thoughts and behaviors. This slight risk seems to appear during the first four weeks of use and should be monitored very carefully by a person's prescribing doctor.

As a result, the FDA requires that all packaging for antidepressants contain a warning label about the possible risk of suicidal thoughts and behaviors in children and teens. The agency also recommends the close monitoring of children and teens during the first month of treatment for sudden changes in behavior, such as highly active behavior or speech, or for depression symptoms that worsen. These behaviors should be reported to a person's regular doctor or psychiatrist as soon as possible. In general, though, the FDA states that the benefits of using antidepressants for children and teens definitely outweigh the possible risks.

Antidepressants for Treating Other Problems

Doctors may prescribe antidepressants for disorders besides depression. These include phobias or anxiety disorders, eating disorders, obsessive-compulsive disorder (OCD), attention deficit hyperactive disorder (ADHD), and significant sleep problems like insomnia.

Severe phobia, panic, or anxiety disorders can interfere with everyday life. Phobias are severe fears about situations or things. For example, you might refuse to leave your house for fear of open or public places, especially those from which escape could be difficult. Some teens might be painfully shy or are always anxious and worried. Panic disorders are conditions in which your fear or anxiety is so strong that it gets in the way of functioning and enjoying life. Panic attacks can be scary. You may have breathing trouble, a racing heartbeat, trembling, dizziness, or a fear of losing control or dying. People who are extremely anxious may also have frequent headaches, upset stomach, or nausea.

The most common teen eating disorders are anorexia ner-vosa (self-starvation), binge eating (cycles of constantly overeating), and bulimia (overeating and vomiting). These dis-orders are fairly common in adolescents, unfortunately, and require medical attention as soon as they are recognized.

Some teens have OCD. Obsessions are constant, reoccurring, and unwanted thoughts or ideas that keep people from thinking about other things. People with obsessions may have extreme fears of harm and may obsess that they will get a deadly disease, for example. Compulsions are urgent, repeated, and irresistible behaviors like washing your hands over and over or checking your schoolwork thirty times for fear that you missed answering a question.

Children or teens with ADHD typically have short attention spans. They have difficulty concentrating or focusing, and they are usually restless. They can often feel frustrated and upset, and they may cause problems in school.

Benefits of Antidepressants

Antidepressants are often an important part of treatment for people of all ages. Teens often receive psychotherapy (talk therapy) along with an antidepressant, since this combined approach usually produces better results. Treatment with anti-depressants lifts depression and reduces or eliminates suicidal thinking and behavior. In addition, antidepressants can help teens better communicate about their depression and get the help they need.

Myths and Facts

 Antidepressants are addictive.
Fact: ➤ Antidepressants are not addictive or habit-forming.

 If you take antidepressants, your personality will change.
Fact: ➤ Antidepressants do not change one's personality. They lift the symptoms of depression so that people can experience the range of normal moods.

 Antidepressants are "happy pills" or "happy drugs."
Fact: ➤ Antidepressants are not chemically related to drugs like amphetamines ("uppers") or to illegal drugs that cause users to initially feel happy. Antidepressants help you feel like your normal self. If some teens who are not depressed take antidepressants, they may feel sick. Most, though, will feel no effects.

two

WHAT IS DEPRESSION?

Depression is a mental illness that requires treatment. If you are depressed, your negative feelings and thoughts dominate your everyday life. This can affect your mood and your behavior at school, in the community, and at home.

Depression is not a sign that people are weak, crazy, or lack character or courage. It is a medical condition. The most common complaint of people who seek counseling is that of feeling depressed.

Teens and Depression

When depression occurs, your brain and body do not work well together. Your brain may stop sending some messages to your body about sleep, movement, eating, and so on. Simple activities like getting out of bed in the morning, combing your hair, or

Some teens who are depressed feel unhappy and sad, lose interest in friends, and may avoid or withdraw from people.

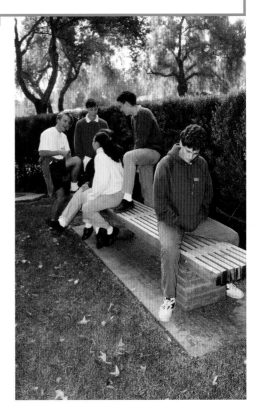

taking a shower may seem impossible.

Symptoms of depression vary for each teen. Some teens may feel deeply sad, hopeless, powerless, empty, or full of despair. Their thoughts stay on a negative track. Many lose interest in activities and hobbies that once were fun. Teens often have difficulty making decisions, concentrating, or thinking. They may have difficulty completing schoolwork. Some teens cry or sleep a lot, while others sleep very little. They may drop all their friends and find new friends who use alcohol and illegal drugs. Other teens withdraw from friends and family because they feel isolated from everyone.

If their painful feelings from depression go untreated for long periods of time, some teens become at increased risk for suicidal behavior and even suicide. The main cause of suicide is depression. According to the National Institute of Mental Health, suicide is the third leading cause of death in teens.

Teens who are depressed may act differently from adults who are depressed. Teens are more likely to be angry, aggressive, irritable, or act out. They tend to sleep and eat more than usual, and they may also have more headaches, stomachaches, back-aches, and other aches and pains that never seem to improve. Other warning signs that teens may be depressed are a drop in grades, skipping school, or quitting school entirely.

Causes of Depression

Researchers are not certain why depression develops in some people. Some think that depression occurs when chemical imbalances in the brain cause low levels of certain neurotrans-mitters. How the body produces and breaks down these neurotransmitters inside and outside of neurons in the brain may be linked to developing depression. In addition, how a pro-tein in the brain called p11 interacts with serotonin may cause some people to develop depression. Other researchers believe that genes are the main factor. You may have a tendency to become depressed because you inherited one or more genes from a parent. Several genes working together may create an increased chance of developing depression. Other researchers think your environment, emotions, or coping skills are the major factors in causing depression. Teens who cope with stress in healthy ways have a lesser chance of developing depression. Many experts think that several (or all) of these factors play an important role.

Risk Factors

Anything that increases a person's chance of having a disease is called a risk factor. Having one or more risk factors does not necessarily mean that you will develop depression. One risk factor is family history. If a family member experiences depression or commits suicide, you may be at higher risk of developing depression. Other risk factors are stressful or painful events, such as when a good friend moves away, a parent dies, or frequent family problems.

Teens may struggle with unrealistic school, social, or family expectations. Constantly trying to live up to these expectations can cause them to feel resentful, angry, powerless, or exhausted. Depression can result. When things go wrong, some teens overreact and may feel that life is not fair or that they are unlucky. Teens who have highly negative feelings and thoughts or low self-confidence seem to have an increased chance of developing depression.

Alcohol and illegal drug use are also risk factors. Some teens who are depressed use alcohol and illegal drugs to try to reduce their pain or sadness. However, alcohol or drug use generally makes depression worse.

Having a physical illness like cancer or heart disease can make daily life difficult, which is stressful and may lead to depression. Some medications may cause depression, such as certain medicines that control high blood pressure. Sometimes, depression is just one of the features of an illness like Alzheimer's disease. Other risk factors for depression include being poor and female. The Agency for Healthcare Research

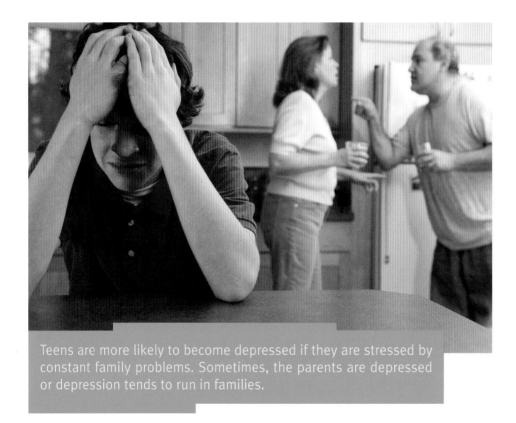

Teens are more likely to become depressed if they are stressed by constant family problems. Sometimes, the parents are depressed or depression tends to run in families.

and Quality reports that almost 6 percent of teens between the ages of thirteen and eighteen are depressed, and depression is more common in girls than boys. According to the Substance Abuse and Mental Health Services Administration, teens who have had one episode of depression are at risk of having another episode within five years.

Types of Depression

Your life can feel overwhelming at times. During your teen years, you take on new responsibilities, such as driving and having a part-time job. You have new challenges, such as adapting to changes in your body, learning to separate from your parents, and figuring out your needs and goals. You might feel unhappy or sad sometimes, or you might feel stressed. However, most teens successfully cope with their ups and downs. They do not feel down for long periods of time. A temporary state of feeling sad, unhappy, or blue is not considered a depression disorder.

Depression that consistently persists for more than two weeks and affects your mind and body in negative ways, though, is considered a possible disorder. There are different types of depression.

Depression

Depression is a medical illness. It affects how you think and behave, and it can cause emotional and physical problems. Depression interferes with your ability to study, eat, sleep, and have fun. Your decision-making, learning, concentration, and problem-solving skills are also affected. If you have depression, you feel excessively sad for more than two weeks. You sleep too much or too little, gain or lose weight because your appetite changes, and lose interest in activities that you once enjoyed. You may feel empty, worthless, and helpless. You may also feel restless or unable to concentrate. Some teens may have only one episode of depression in their lifetime. Others may have repeated episodes of depression throughout their lives

Dysthymia

Dysthymia is a mild form of depression that lasts two or more years. If dysthymia starts in childhood, it can often last longer than two years. This disorder can make it difficult for you to remember better times or enjoy your life, although you may have occasional mood lifts. People with dysthymia may have one or more episodes of depression during their lifetime. Dysthymia occurs more often in females than males. According to the National Institutes of Health, dysthymia affects up to 5 percent of people in the United States.

Seasonal Affective Disorder

People with seasonal affective disorder (SAD) feel sad and tired in the winter, when the hours of daylight decrease. During these winter months, you may gain weight, sleep too much, or withdraw from friends and social activities. Your sad feelings typically lift in the spring and summer. With more hours of sunlight, you feel like yourself and can enjoy your friends and regular activities again. The American Academy of Family Physicians estimates that about five hundred thousand people in the United States may have SAD. This disorder can often be treated successfully with light therapy.

Bipolar Disorder

Bipolar disorder is not as common as other forms of depression, but it can be a serious illness. People with bipolar disorder have radical emotional changes and mood swings, from manic "highs" to depressive "lows." During manic periods, you may not sleep much, have great energy, feel very happy, and think you can do anything. You may talk too much and too fast, make many impossible plans, and try to squeeze in lots of activities. You might be impulsive, spend money freely, or take serious risks like abusing

Seasonal affective disorder (SAD) is a depression following a lack of light and warmth, particularly during the winter. Light therapy can help. This light therapy box gives off bright light that mimics natural outdoor light.

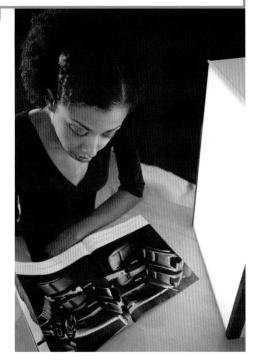

alcohol and illegal drugs. Your extreme mood swings can last for weeks or months, and they can affect you, your family, and your friends. Then the depressive symptoms take over, and you feel sad, unmotivated, and withdrawn. The cycles of highs and lows can last for weeks or even months.

Although bipolar disorder typically starts in the teen years or early adulthood, it can start in childhood. If untreated, it usually becomes worse over time. During the depressive period, some people get so low that they become suicidal and may even take their life.

Whatever type of depression you may have, getting diagnosed is the first step to getting treatment and support.

three

HOW IS DEPRESSION DETECTED AND DIAGNOSED?

Depression can affect anyone of any age, gender, religion, or race. A health professional can officially determine whether or not someone has depression. Once diagnosed, this disorder is usually highly treatable.

Warning Signs of Depression

If you are depressed, you may have some of the following signs for two or more weeks:

- Feeling sad most of the time
- Unable to have fun
- Having no energy; feeling very tired
- Increased appetite or loss of appetite
- Oversleeping or difficulty sleeping

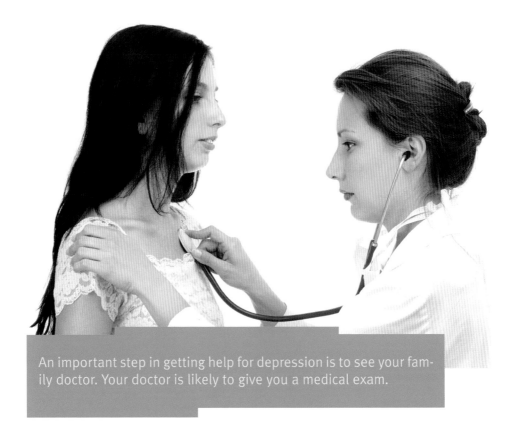

An important step in getting help for depression is to see your family doctor. Your doctor is likely to give you a medical exam.

- Irritability, anger, worry, agitation (extreme restlessness)
- Feeling guilty, worthless, or overly anxious
- Difficulty concentrating or making decisions
- Unexplained aches and pains
- Spending less and less time with friends
- Frequent thoughts of suicide or death

If you persistently experience five or more of these symptoms for more than two weeks, or if any of these symptoms interferes with your daily life, seek help. You can read about

During the mania phase of bipolar disorder, teens may spend money recklessly and make other odd decisions quickly, sometimes with serious consequences.

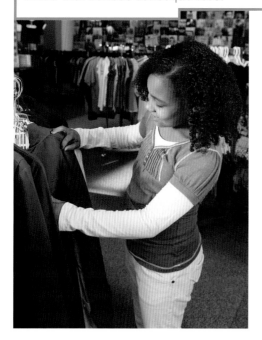

the many people who can help you in chapter 4.

Warning Signs of Bipolar Disorder

People who have bipolar disorder experience mood shifts that disrupt their everyday activities. The signs of the depressive phase of this illness are similar to those of depression. The signs of mania include the following:

- High energy, happiness, and activity
- Extreme irritability; aggressive behavior
- Increased moving and talking
- Decreased need for sleep, but doesn't feel tired
- Grand ideas; feels very self-important
- Racing speech and racing thoughts
- Impulsive; poor judgment (like spending a lot of money); easy to distract
- Reckless, rude, or annoying behavior

- Does not think there is a problem with extreme behavior or emotions

If you think you may cycle between mania and depression, talk to someone who can help you.

If You Think You Are Depressed

Depression requires treatment. You might think that you can "snap out of it" because you can beat your depression through inner strength, or your friends or parents tell you to cheer up or stop moping. You can't, since depression does not go away on its own. Some teens might not seek help because they think their friends will see them as different, weak, cowardly, or crazy. Or you may fear that your friends will make fun of you or reject you if they know your true feelings. Some people bottle up their feelings and don't tell anyone how sad, hopeless, or angry they feel.

It's OK to talk to someone you trust about how you feel. You might want to start with a parent, guardian, or friend's parent. Perhaps you may feel comfortable talking with a teacher or coach. Other people you can talk with are your school counselor, nurse, social worker, or psychologist. Religious leaders or counselors are trained in mental health issues and can be helpful. You may want to talk in person with your family doctor.

To find a mental health specialist, ask friends or family members for a recommendation. Your school counselor may be a good resource, too. You can also do your own research to find a mental health specialist. Every state has mental health resources. Look in your local telephone book or on the Internet for places that offer mental health services. Call and ask to talk to a mental health professional at your local mental health center, hotline, crisis center, hospital, or clinic. Or check with a state or national professional organization to find local mental health specialists. The federal government provides a mental health services locator for every state at http://www.mentalhealth.samhsa.gov/databases.

If You Feel Suicidal

If you are thinking about suicide, it is very important to tell someone immediately. You can call a suicide crisis line for teens at any time, seven days a week. These trained people will listen to you and discuss your feelings and problems. You may also want to talk to an adult you trust. If you might really take your own life, call 911 or get to your local hospital emergency room right away. Talking about your suicidal thoughts or plans may be scary and painful. By opening up and being honest with someone you trust, you can get help.

Getting Diagnosed by a Doctor

Getting diagnosed by a professional is the next step in getting help for your depression. You might start with an appointment with your family doctor. Your doctor may evaluate your physical and mental health. He or she may ask questions about your medical history and symptoms of depression. Questions can include when your symptoms started, how long they have lasted, and how severe they are. Your doctor will want to know about prior episodes of depression, including treatment. Be honest when

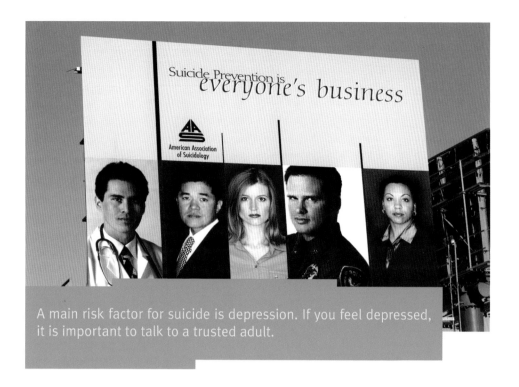

A main risk factor for suicide is depression. If you feel depressed, it is important to talk to a trusted adult.

answering questions about alcohol or illegal drug use and whether you are thinking about death or suicide.

Tell your doctor of any prescription medication, over-the-counter medicine, or supplements you are taking. He or she will also record your family medical history and note any family history of depression or suicide. You will have a physical exam. Laboratory tests will be run. Some medications and medical conditions, such as chronic virus infections or thyroid disorders, can cause symptoms similar to those of depression. Your doctor can evaluate these possibilities from your exam and lab tests.

After your doctor has analyzed your information, you will find out the results. You may have a medical disorder or illness. With proper treatment for your medical problem, your depression may lift. If depression appears to be your main problem, your doctor will probably refer you to a mental health professional for evaluation and treatment.

Getting Diagnosed by a Mental Health Specialist

Mental health professionals evaluate and treat people for depression. Some specialize in working with teens or children. Mental health specialists who conduct assessments (evaluations) include psychiatrists, psychologists, and social workers. An assessment is like an interview between you and your mental health professional. It can take two to three hours and may require one or more office visits.

The mental health specialist will ask you about your concerns and causes of stress. If your family doctor has not evaluated you, the mental health expert will ask you about your medical history, family medical history, medications, and supplements. You will also talk about your family, friends, school, and more. You might take several tests about your mental state. The mental health expert may also interview your parents or guardians. To interview other family members, counselors, or teachers, the professional will need permission from your parents or guardians, and he or she should ask you for your permission. Results from the laboratory tests will be included in your assessment. The mental health specialist will then evaluate your information and arrive at a diagnosis.

Health professionals usually base a diagnosis of depression on whether or not you have certain symptoms that are

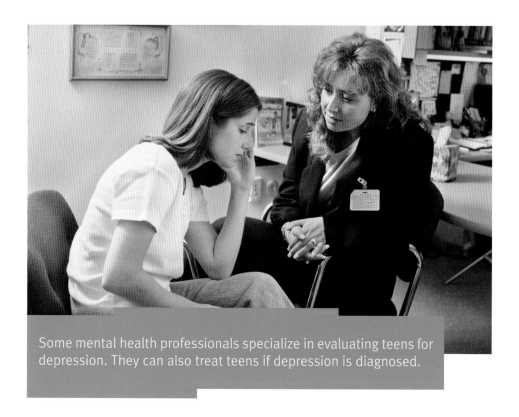

Some mental health professionals specialize in evaluating teens for depression. They can also treat teens if depression is diagnosed.

listed in the American Psychiatric Association's *Diagnostic and Statistical Manual of Mental Disorders, Fourth Edition, Text Revision*, also known as the *DSM IV-TR*. This book lists and describes hundreds of mental illnesses. Your diagnosis depends on the number of symptoms you have, how severe they are, and how long they have lasted. For the symptoms of depression given in the *DSM-IV-TR*, see the warning signs at the beginning of this chapter.

Health professionals also use the *DSM IV-TR* to diagnose bipolar disorder. For the symptoms of bipolar disorder given in the *DSM-IV-TR*, see the warning signs at the beginning of this chapter.

HOW IS DEPRESSION TREATED?

Once you are diagnosed with a type of depression, your mental health specialist will discuss a treatment plan with you and your parents. Bring up any concerns or questions, and get answers before starting your treatment.

Your mental health professional will recommend a treatment plan for you. This may include reading helpful books and pamphlets, having regular therapy, taking medication, or being treated with therapy and medication together. The goal of your treatment plan is to reduce or eliminate your depression and prevent a reoccurrence.

Types of Therapists

Mental health professionals who can provide therapy are psychiatrists, clinical psychologists, clinical social workers, and counselors of various types. They often work in

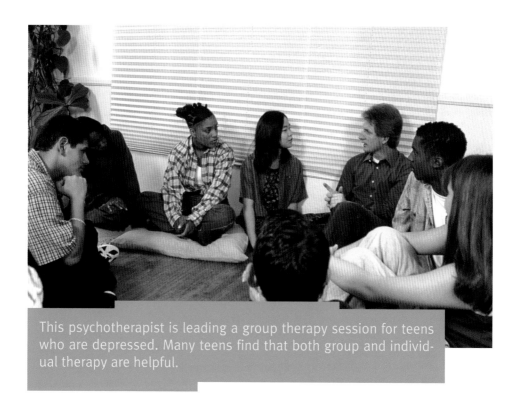

This psychotherapist is leading a group therapy session for teens who are depressed. Many teens find that both group and individual therapy are helpful.

hospitals, clinics, or private offices. Most state governments have an office that oversees the licensing of mental health professionals, and each state has specific requirements for licensed therapists. Here are some of the types of therapists who provide treatment for mental health problems.

Psychiatrists

Psychiatrists are medical doctors (MDs) who have completed additional medical training in mental health disorders. They specialize in diagnosing and treating mental, emotional, and behavioral disorders. Psychiatrists can prescribe medication, order laboratory tests, conduct assessments, and evaluate and treat mental disorders. They use a variety of therapies to help people.

Family Doctors

Some family doctors are trained in psychotherapy and can provide counseling. They can also write prescriptions for medications.

Clinical Psychologists

These psychologists test, diagnose, and treat emotional and behavioral disorders through various psychotherapies. They cannot prescribe medications. Clinical psychologists have a graduate degree in psychology (Ph.D. or Psy.D.). Each state determines the training required to become a psychologist.

Clinical Social Workers

Clinical social workers have a master's degree in social work (MSW), and additional training and experience in diagnosing and treating emotional disorders. They work in schools, mental health clinics, family service agencies, and in private practices.

Counselors

Many kinds of counselors work with teens. School counselors usually have a master's degree and can help with emotional and educational matters. Addiction counselors have special training and certification to help people who abuse alcohol or other drugs. Religious counselors receive training to help people with mental, social, and marriage problems.

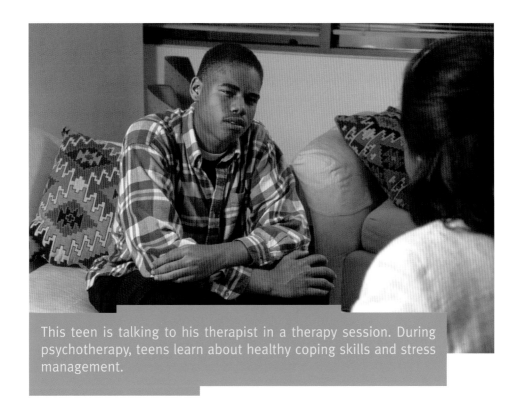

This teen is talking to his therapist in a therapy session. During psychotherapy, teens learn about healthy coping skills and stress management.

Your Therapist

You may want to meet with a few therapists before choosing one. Ask about their training, certification, and experience. Choose a therapist who is respectful of you and gives you hope that you can feel better.

Therapy sessions may be private, with just you and the therapist. Therapy can also involve your family, especially if you request it. Therapy may also be a support group of teens who have depression. Talk with your therapist about your choices and what to do if something is not working for you.

What you and your therapist talk about during your sessions is private. However, therapists have a professional responsibility to protect you. For example, they are required by law to break your confidentiality (trust) if you threaten to kill or harm yourself or others.

Psychotherapy (Talk Therapy)

During psychotherapy, you have regular sessions with your therapist. Each session may last between thirty and sixty minutes, and occur once or twice a week. Psychotherapy usually runs ten to twenty weeks, sometimes longer, depending on your needs and what your family's health insurance allows. During your sessions, you talk with your therapist about your feelings, behaviors, and problems regarding relationships, mental health issues, or emotional issues.

At first, you may feel uncomfortable discussing your feelings. Give therapy some time. It may not be easy to talk about thoughts and feelings that you may have hidden. Psychotherapy can be intense. Sometimes, you may feel upset or even cry during or after sessions.

Through therapy, you learn possible causes for your depression. You identify unhealthy behaviors and negative thoughts, and you learn how to change them. Your therapist can help you find better ways to solve problems and cope with everyday changes. After going through psychotherapy, teens often feel happier and more in control of their lives. They learn new and effective ways to deal with their problems.

Types of Psychotherapy for Treating Depression

Several types of psychotherapy work well in treating depression. Cognitive behavioral therapy (CBT) is the most common type of therapy for depression. During CBT, you focus on your thoughts (cognition) and how they determine your behavior. You identify negative beliefs and behaviors, and you replace them with positive, healthy ones. In addition, you learn how to set realistic goals and discover what you want from life.

Interpersonal therapy and psychodynamic psychotherapy are other commonly used therapies. Through interpersonal therapy, you learn to understand and work through troubled personal relationships that may cause your depression or make it worse.

Psychodynamic psychotherapy helps you look at your conscious and unconscious emotional issues. By doing so, you can better understand your emotional responses to difficult relationships. Sometimes, teens repeat patterns of relating to others that do not work well or are unhealthy. Psychodynamic psychotherapy can help you change how you see and interact with people and relationships.

Psychopharmacological therapy, or combination therapy, is treatment using both talk therapy and antidepressant medication. Antidepressants help lift your depression so that you feel happier and meet the challenges of each day. By relieving your depression, you can better communicate your thoughts and feelings, and improve your outlook on life.

Treating Depression with Antidepressants

Your psychiatrist or doctor may prescribe an antidepressant. Dozens of antidepressants are available to treat depression. The FDA has approved only fluoxetine for treating depression in teens, although there are other similar medications commonly prescribed for teens. Fluoxetine is a selective serotonin reuptake inhibitor (SSRI). Doctors usually prescribe SSRIs for teens. Doctors can also use their judgment to prescribe other medications that may be effective but haven't been approved yet by the FDA to treat depression in children and teens. This legal and common practice is called off-label use.

Each type of antidepressant works differently. To determine which antidepressant may work best for you, your doctor will analyze your assessment and diagnosis. Your assessment includes your symptoms, family history of depression, medications that have helped family members with depression, and other conditions that you may have.

In addition to an antidepressant, your doctor may prescribe other medications to treat your depression or other mood disorders. Sometimes, your doctor may combine two or more antidepressants or other medications if your symptoms do not significantly improve while taking one medicine.

Recall that an antidepressant usually takes from two to four weeks before it affects your mood. You may notice that your thoughts are less negative and clearer, your sleep is better, and you feel better. An antidepressant can take six to eight weeks

Antidepressant medications can be useful in treating depression. The medications typically take a few weeks to work and are not addictive.

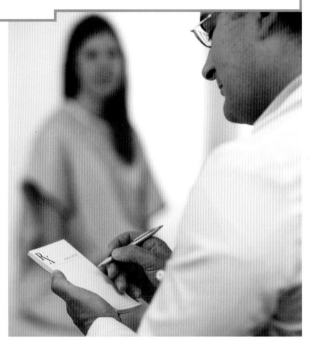

until it is fully effective, though, so try to remain patient. Before starting an antidepressant, ask your doctor about the possible side effects and what to report immediately.

The various antidepressants usually have about the same effectiveness. What works well for one family member tends to work well for other family members. However, no one SSRI is effective for every person. Switching medications may prove effective for you if the first doesn't work. You may need to try more than one or two antidepressants. Some teens find that it can take several months or even a year or more to find an antidepressant that works well. Keep trying! Scientists are researching how to increase the speed at which antidepressants can work effectively. In the future, you may know within two to three days how an antidepressant is working for you.

Ten Great Questions to Ask Your Doctor

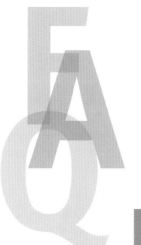

1 What treatment do you advise for my depression?

2 How soon will I start feeling better after taking this antidepressant?

3 What should I do if I don't feel better?

4 How long will it take to feel the full benefit of this antidepressant?

5 What are the common side effects of this antidepressant, and how should I deal with them?

6 What side effects are serious enough that I should contact you immediately?

7 What foods or medications can interact with this antidepressant?

8 What should I do if I miss a dose of an antidepressant?

9 How long will I need to take an antidepressant?

10 What should I do if I'm having suicidal thoughts?

part
five

WHAT ARE
THE TYPES OF
ANTIDEPRESSANTS?

The most commonly prescribed types of antidepressants are selective serotonin reuptake inhibitors (SSRIs) and serotonin and norepinephrine reuptake inhibitors (SNRIs). Doctors prescribe SSRIs more than any other type of antidepressant for teens and adults. If SSRIs don't work, they may prescribe an SNRI. Their last choice would be antidepressants that work differently from how SSRIs and SNRIs work, such as tricyclic antidepressants (TCAs) and monoamine oxidase inhibitors (MAOIs). TCAs and MAOIs are older types of antidepressants. Doctors still prescribe them for various problems, although their side effects tend to be more significant. For this reason, they are seldom prescribed for children or teens.

Antidepressants and other medications have generic names. Many have one or more brand names. The

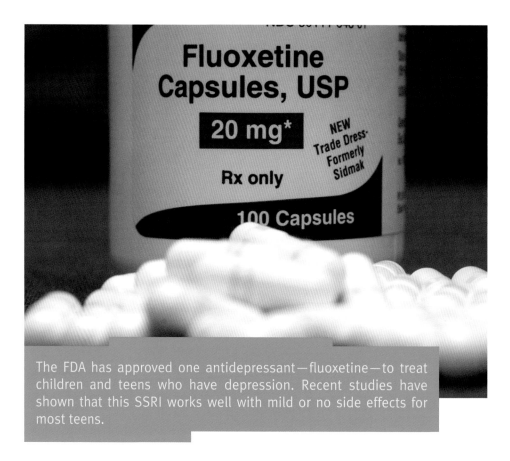

The FDA has approved one antidepressant—fluoxetine—to treat children and teens who have depression. Recent studies have shown that this SSRI works well with mild or no side effects for most teens.

generic name is the chemical name of a medication. The brand name is the advertised name of a medication that a drug company sells. Generic drugs are chemically identical to the brand-name versions, and they're just as safe and effective. Generic medications cost less than the brand names. When writing the name of a medication, the generic name comes first, followed by the brand name in parentheses.

Antidepressants are not usually prescribed for people with bipolar disorder, since they can bring on a manic episode.

Instead, many health professionals prescribe lithium or other medications to help even out the extreme mood swings of bipolar disorder.

Selective Serotonin Reuptake Inhibitors (SSRIs)

You may know the generic and brand names of some SSRIs: fluoxetine (Prozac), sertraline (Zoloft), paroxetine (Paxil), fluvoxamine (Luvox), citalopram (Celexa), and escitalopram (Lexapro). Recall that SSRIs increase the level of serotonin in your brain. This neurotransmitter affects the regions of your brain that involve mood, emotions, sex drive, and aggression. SSRIs slow the neurons from taking up serotonin. This causes more serotonin to be available, and depression lifts.

SSRIs are common medications. According to Verispan, a health care reporting agency, more than twenty-eight million prescriptions of sertraline (Zoloft) and more than twenty-two million prescriptions of fluoxetine (Prozac) were filled in the United States in 2007. Millions of people take SSRIs to relieve their depression. Doctors may also prescribe these medications to treat anxiety, social phobia, obsessive compulsive disorder, eating disorders, and other disorders.

The main side effects of SSRIs are mild nausea and diarrhea. Other side effects may include dry mouth, headaches, feeling nervous or jittery, restlessness, increased sweating, appetite problems, feeling drowsy, sleep problems, and rash. People may notice some changes in sexual functions.

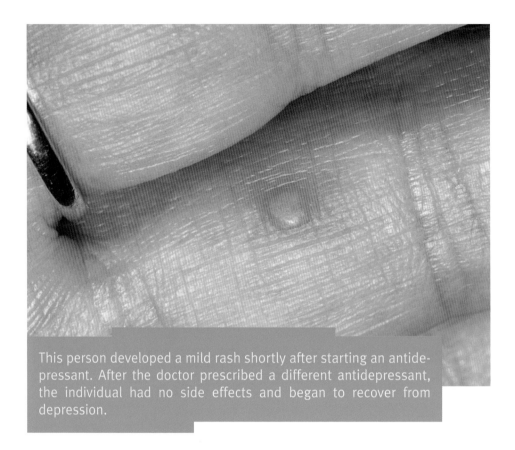

This person developed a mild rash shortly after starting an antidepressant. After the doctor prescribed a different antidepressant, the individual had no side effects and began to recover from depression.

Serotonin syndrome can occur if SSRIs interact with other antidepressants, antihistamines (medications for allergy relief), and some other medications. This rare, but serious, condition requires medical treatment as soon as possible. Serotonin syndrome results from extremely high levels of serotonin in the brain. It can occur when an SSRI interacts with an MAOI antidepressant. The syndrome can also be triggered if SSRIs are combined with some prescription pain relievers for migraines or herbal supplements that affect serotonin levels, such as

St. John's wort. Signs of serotonin syndrome are confusion, fever, extreme agitation, sweating, high blood pressure, fast heartbeat, nausea, vomiting, and hallucinations (imaginary sights, sounds, and smells that are believed to be real). Some people may have trembling or seizures or even slip into a coma.

Selective Serotonin and Norepinephrine Reuptake Inhibitors (SNRIs)

If SSRIs don't work, doctors may prescribe another type of antidepressant, such as serotonin and norepinephrine reuptake inhibitors (SNRIs). Two SNRIs are venlafaxine (Effexor) and duloxetine (Cymbalta). SNRIs slow down the reuptake of both serotonin and norepinephrine. Common side effects are nausea, headaches, sleep problems, feeling nervous or jittery, rashes, and appetite problems. Serotonin syndrome can result if an SNRI is combined with other medications or herbal supplements, such as St. John's wort.

Wellbutrin

In addition to SSRIs and SNRIs, some other antidepressants may be good choices. Unlike other antidepressants, bupropion (Wellbutrin) affects the neurotransmitters norepinephrine and dopamine. Both neurotransmitters affect mood and emotion. Like other antidepressants, Wellbutrin can take three to four weeks or more to reach its full effect. Side effects may include headaches, nausea, vomiting, dry mouth, constipation, and mild tremors. If you've had seizures, or if you have an eating disorder, you may have a slight risk of bupropion triggering a seizure. This medication is also used to help people with seasonal affective disorder (SAD).

Remeron

Mirtazapine (Remeron) affects norepinephrine and serotonin differently than other antidepressants. It works by blocking the receptors that inhibit the release of these neurotransmitters. This causes the release of norepinephrine and serotonin, and the resulting increased levels of the neurotransmitters can improve mood. Side effects of Remeron can include dry mouth, feeling dizzy or light-headed, increased appetite, thirst, muscle or joint aches, constipation, and weight gain. Some people may see a rise in their cholesterol level, which may increase their chance of having a stroke.

Tricyclic Antidepressants (TCAs)

Tricyclic antidepressants (TCAs) derive their name from their composition of three fused rings of carbon atoms. They inhibit the reuptake of serotonin and norepinephrine by neurons. TCAs bind other cell surface receptors, though, and this blockade can cause many side effects. Some side effects include dry mouth, nausea, constipation, blurred vision, increased heartbeat, headaches, and sensitivity to light. People may feel drowsy, weak, dizzy, or confused. Others may have difficulty urinating and notice some changes in sexual functions. If very high doses are taken, people could have irregular heartbeats, which can be fatal. People should avoid eating grapefruit while on TCAs. Grapefruit can cause extremely high and dangerous levels of the medication to remain in the body.

Monoamine Oxidase Inhibitors (MAOIs)

Doctors seldom prescribe monoamine oxidase inhibitors (MAOIs) for teens. If you take a MAOI, you must follow a restricted diet and avoid many types of medication. MAOIs can be effective at lifting mood for certain people. Doctors typically consider these antidepressants only when other classes of anti-depressants don't work. MAOIs inhibit the activity of the enzymes that break down some neurotransmitters, including serotonin, norepinephrine, and dopamine. As the levels of these neurotransmitters increase, depression is relieved. The side effects of MAOIs are similar to those of tricyclic antidepressants. They can also cause weight gain, muscle twitches, trembling, and low blood pressure.

MAOIs can interact with food and medications that contain high levels of tyramine. This chemical influences blood pressure. People taking MAOIs must avoid many cheeses, pickled foods, chocolate, figs, certain meats and beans, and soy sauce. The interaction of high levels of tyramine in these foods and a MAOI can cause blood pressure to skyrocket, which can lead to a stroke. Ask your doctor for a list of foods and beverages to avoid.

MAOIs can also cause serious reactions if taken with other antidepressants and some prescription pain relievers. They can also interact with some over-the-counter medicines and herbal supplements, such as St. John's wort. Never take MAOIs with SSRIs due to the high risk of serotonin syndrome.

Side Effects of Antidepressants

The list of possible side effects of SSRIs, SNRIs, and other anti-depressants may seem scary. Side effects vary widely from person to person. Some teens experience no side effects. Most experience only minor discomfort when starting and using SSRIs, SNRIs, and other antidepressants, such as Wellbutrin and Remeron. Many teens find that side effects lessen or disappear by the second month of use.

Often, teens with depression find that taking an antidepressant and having therapy stabilizes their mood and helps relieve symptoms of depression. You can also take steps on your own to treat your depression and increase your chance of avoiding it in the future.

HOW WILL TAKING ANTIDEPRESSANTS AFFECT MY LIFESTYLE?

Agreeing to use an antidepressant is a strong step forward in dealing with your depression. Unless you tell your friends, they probably won't know you're taking an antidepressant. They will notice that you have more energy, and you are more positive and fun. As your depression lifts and you learn effective ways to handle your emotional problems through therapy, you can take other steps to feel better.

Taking Antidepressants

When you get your prescription from a pharmacy, you will also receive printed information about your antidepressant. Be sure to read this information. It includes the name

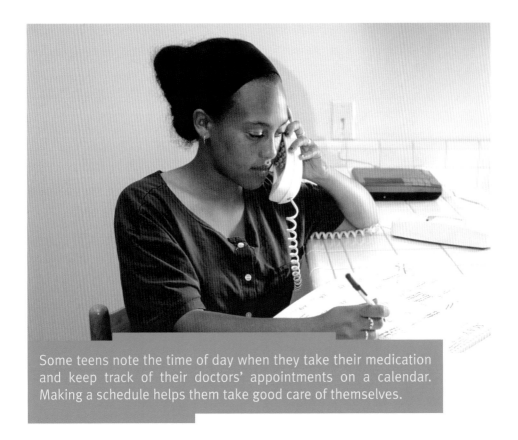

Some teens note the time of day when they take their medication and keep track of their doctors' appointments on a calendar. Making a schedule helps them take good care of themselves.

of your medication and what it looks like, instructions on using it, what to avoid while taking it, information your doctor must know before you begin taking it, and its possible side effects. You will also learn what severe side effects to report to your doctor immediately.

The antidepressant that you try first may work fine for you. Or it may take some time to find an antidepressant that works for you. Sometimes, an SSRI might work for a while, but then side effects begin, such as feeling jittery or daytime sleepiness. Tell your doctor if your antidepressant is not helping. Your doctor may increase your dose, start you at a low dose, and then gradually increase the dose. Or he or she may switch you to a different antidepressant.

Ask your doctor what to do if you miss a dose. To help maintain an optimal level of the antidepressant in your body, take your medication about the same time every day. Make a schedule and post it in your day planner, in your room, or on the refrigerator. You can also associate it with something you do every day, such as brushing your teeth or eating breakfast. Also write down your appointments with your doctor or therapist. And write down appointments for laboratory tests that your doctor will use to monitor your body functions.

Ask your school nurse, or read your school handbook, to find out if your school has a policy about prescription medications. If you take your antidepressant during school hours, you may need a note from your parents or guardians about your medication. You will probably store and take your antidepressant at the office of the school nurse or counselor.

Coping with Side Effects of Antidepressants

Side effects are usually a minor discomfort for most people. For example, you may have dry mouth. Try drinking six to eight glasses of water a day, chewing gum, or sucking ice chips. Drinking plenty of water will also help ease diarrhea. For constipation, eat more bran cereals, whole grains, fruits, and vegetables. Blurred vision often passes quickly. However, if

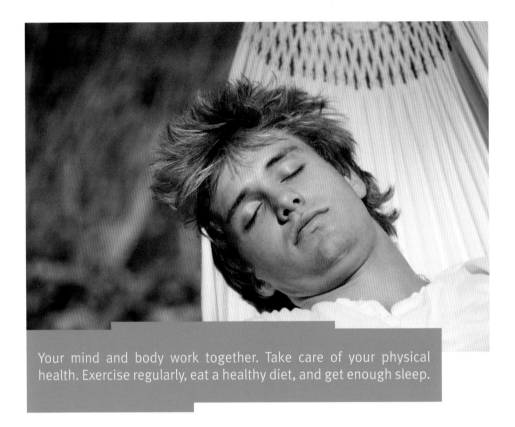

Your mind and body work together. Take care of your physical health. Exercise regularly, eat a healthy diet, and get enough sleep.

your eyes feel dry or irritated, talk to your doctor about soothing eye drops.

If you have nausea or an upset stomach, take your antidepressant with food or try eating smaller meals four to six times a day. Avoid greasy and highly spiced foods. If your nausea continues, ask your doctor for an extended or controlled-release form of your antidepressant. If your appetite is increasing and you are eating more, head off weight gain by cutting out sweets, sodas, chips, and fast foods, which often contain large amounts of fat, salt, and sugar.

Feeling drowsy during the day is a side effect that usually disappears after awhile. Don't drive when you're feeling sleepy. If you continue to feel drowsy or tired, talk with your doctor. Taking your antidepressant at bedtime, rather than in the morning, may eliminate sleepiness during the day. A brief nap (lasting about ten to twenty minutes) in the morning or early afternoon may help. So may a brisk walk. Some people, though, may feel agitated, restless, or anxious. Tell your doctor if these sides effect don't disappear.

Insomnia could be a side effect. Consuming caffeine in the afternoon or evening may be contributing to your sleep problem. Caffeine is a stimulant that peps people up. Foods and beverages that contain caffeine include coffee, tea, some energy drinks and sodas, sweets with caffeine, some over-the-counter medicines, and chocolate.

Talk to your doctor about any side effects that linger or trouble you. Your doctor may change your dose, prescribe another drug to counter your side effect, or prescribe a different antidepressant.

Going Off of Antidepressants

Most mental health professionals initially recommend that teens continue taking their antidepressant six to nine months, perhaps longer. Discuss with your doctor how long your antidepressant treatment will last. The length of time may also depend on your symptoms. Near your planned end date, talk with your doctor to determine if you should stop taking your antidepressant or continue. If you've had depression in the past, your doctor may recommend that you take long-term medication to help prevent your illness from recurring. Some people may take their antidepressant for years so that their depression doesn't return.

Don't stop taking your antidepressant suddenly, or you may have withdrawal symptoms like nausea, sleep problems, tremors, muscle spasms, or headaches. Some teens might feel anxious, agitated, restless, tired, or dizzy. These symptoms are usually mild and typically last a few days or a few weeks. Your doctor will give you a plan for tapering off your medication, which usually involves taking increasingly smaller doses for one to two months.

Improving Your Lifestyle

Following a healthy lifestyle can help keep your mind and body strong and well. Get enough sleep. Most teens require nine or more hours of sleep every day. Include plenty of whole grains, fruits, and vegetables in your diet. Get regular exercise, prefer-ably every day. Activities like team sports or a brisk walk can lift your spirits, increase oxygen to your brain, and get your heart and blood pumping at a steady rate. Exercise will also help keep your body toned. Find something that you enjoy— jogging, hiking, skiing, biking, swimming, or dancing, for example. Washing your car, raking leaves, or shoveling snow from a driveway is also exercise.

Find ways to express your feelings. Write your thoughts in a journal, draw, or find other creative outlets like photography,

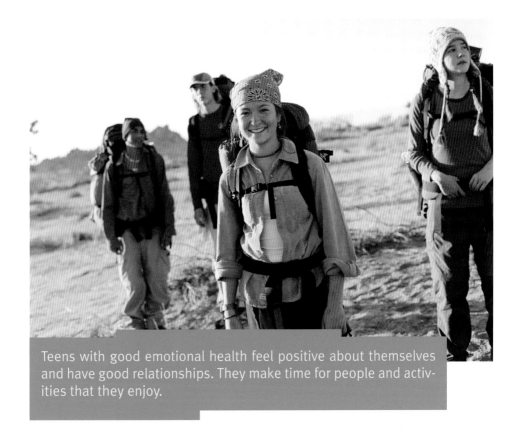

Teens with good emotional health feel positive about themselves and have good relationships. They make time for people and activities that they enjoy.

acting, or playing a musical instrument. Some teens like to sing, dance, paint, make pottery, or write plays or fiction.

Who you spend time with is important. Be with people who are positive, supportive, and encouraging. When you are going through a tough time, you might want to confide in friends, a family member, or a counselor. Make a list of people you can trust to listen to you. You may want to join a support group for teens. Members of the group exchange information and help each other develop healthy ways to cope with problems. Try doing something for someone else. This takes the focus away from you and your feelings. Volunteer your time to a cause you believe in, such as the environment, animal welfare, or supporting a food bank. Even giving someone a compliment makes you and that person feel good.

Develop stress management skills. Managing stress means taking charge of your thoughts and emotions. Deep breathing, muscle relaxation, stretching, and yoga can clear your mind and relax your body. You might enjoy listening to soothing music, watching the clouds roll by, or sipping a cup of herbal tea. Laughing is a great way to relieve stress. Watch a funny movie, or share silly jokes with a friend. Learn to say no so that you don't overextend yourself. If you stretch yourself too thin, it's difficult to stay calm and in charge of yourself.

All of these suggestions can help you build self-confidence and feel better about yourself and your life. You can learn how to make the best of any situation and handle change, both good and bad. You will feel a sense of hope for today and the future.

antidepressant A prescription medication used to treat depression and other disorders, such as panic and eating disorders and anxiety.

anxiety A feeling of unease and distress that may not be related to any particular object or situation.

bipolar disorder A type of mental illness that causes extreme mood swings, from intense excitement and happiness to deep depression; formerly called manic-depressive illness.

cognitive behavioral therapy (CBT) A type of therapy that helps people recognize and change negative patterns of thinking that may contribute to their depression.

depression A period in which a person feels hopeless, sad, and in despair; formerly called clinical depression or major depression.

dopamine A chemical in the brain that affects mood and behavior.

dysthymia A type of mild depression that involves long-lasting symptoms that aren't seriously disabling.

mania A period of extreme excitement and activity, rapidly shifting ideas, and lack of sleep.

monoamine oxidase inhibitors (MAOIs) A class of antide-pressants used to treat depression and other disorders.

neuron A nerve cell.

neurotransmitter A chemical in the brain that carries messages between neurons.

norepinephrine A chemical in the brain that affects mood and behavior.

obsessive compulsive disorder (OCD) A mental disorder in which someone has a distressing set of repetitive thoughts and actions.

psychiatrist A physician specializing in evaluating and treating mental illness.

psychotherapy A treatment that helps people understand their thoughts, feelings, behaviors, and relationships with others.

seasonal affective disorder (SAD) A condition characterized by feeling sad and tired in the winter, when there is little daylight, and then feeling fine in the spring and summer.

selective serotonin reuptake inhibitors (SSRIs) A class of antidepressants used to treat depression and other mental disorders. SSRIs slow the reuptake of serotonin.

serotonin A chemical in the brain that affects mood and behavior.

serotonin and norepinephrine reuptake inhibitors (SNRIs) A class of antidepressants used to treat depression and other mental disorders. SNRIs slow the reuptake of serotonin and norepinephrine.

serotonin syndrome A rare, serious condition caused by very high levels of serotonin.

tricyclic antidepressants (TCAs) A class of antidepressants that are named for their three-ring chemical structure.

withdrawal The unpleasant symptoms that occur when someone suddenly stops taking an antidepressant.

American Academy of Child and Adolescent Psychiatry
3615 Wisconsin Avenue NW
Washington, DC 20016-3007
(202) 966-7300
Web site: http:www.aacap.org
   This nonprofit organization supports and advances child
   and teen psychiatry through research and distribution of
   information.

American Psychological Association
750 First Street NE
Washington, DC 20002-4242
(202) 336-5700
Web site: http://www.apa.org
   This organization provides information about mental
   disorders and offers referrals to psychologists who can
   provide treatment.

Canadian Mental Health Association
8 King Street East, Suite 810
Toronto, ON M5C 1B5
Canada
(416) 484-7750
Web site: http://www.cmha.ca

The Canadian Mental Health Association provides programs for people who have mental illnesses.

Mood Disorders Society of Canada
3-304 Stone Road West, Suite 736
Guelph, ON N1G 4W4
Canada
(519) 824-5565
Web site: http://www.mooddisorderscanada.ca
This society works to improve the quality of life for people affected by depression, bipolar disorder, and related disorders.

National Foundation for Depressive Illness, Inc.
P.O. Box 2257
New York, NY 10116
(800) 248-4344
Web site: http://www.depression.org
This organization is a good resource for information on depression. Its Web site provides links to most of the major associations dealing with depression.

National Institute of Mental Health
6001 Executive Boulevard
Room 8184, MSC 9663
Bethesda, MD 20892-9663
(866) 615-6464
Web site: http://www.nimh.nih.gov
This federal agency conducts research on mental health, including the causes, prevention, diagnosis, and treatment of

mental illnesses. It also offers publications on understanding and treating mental illnesses.

National Mental Health Information Center
P.O. Box 2345
Rockville, MD 20847
(800) 789-2647
Web site: http://www.mentalhealth.samhsa.gov
The National Mental Health Information Center provides information about mental health by telephone, Web site, and through more than six hundred publications.

U.S. Food and Drug Administration
5600 Fishers Lane
Rockville, MD 20857-0001
(888) 463-6332
Web site: http://www.fda.gov
This federal agency is charged with protecting the health of the public against unsafe drugs, foods, and cosmetics. It approves the use of prescription medications.

Web Sites

Due to the changing nature of Internet links, Rosen Publishing has developed an online list of Web sites related to the subject of this book. This site is updated regularly. Please use this link to access this list:

http://www.rosenlinks.com/faq/anti

Antidepressants: The Complete Series. Philadelphia, PA:
Mason Crest Publishers, 2008.

Dudley, William. *Antidepressants.* San Diego, CA:
Reference Point Press, 2008.

Dudley, William, ed. *The History of Drugs:
Antidepressants.* Detroit, MI: Greenhaven
Press, 2005.

Dunbar, Katherine Read. *Antidepressants: At Issue.*
Detroit, MI: Greenhaven Press, 2005.

Hipp, Earl. *Fighting Invisible Tigers: A Stress Management
Guide for Teens.* Minneapolis, MN: Free Spirit
Publishing, 2008.

Hunter, David. *Antidepressants and Advertising.*
Philadelphia, PA: Mason Crest Publishers, 2007.

Hyde, Margaret O., and John F. Setaro. *Drugs 101: An
Overview for Teens.* Minneapolis, MN: Twenty-First
Century Books, 2003.

Kleiman, Andrew. *Antidepressants and Their Side Effects:
Managing the Risks.* Philadelphia, PA: Mason Crest
Publishers, 2007.

Koellhoffer, Tara. *Prozac and Other Antidepressants.*
Philadelphia, PA: Chelsea House Publishers, 2008.

LeVert, Suzanne. *The Facts About Antidepressants.* New
York, NY: Marshall Cavendish, 2007.

Mitchell, E. Siobhan, and David J. Triggle. *Antidepressants.* Philadelphia, PA: Chelsea House Publishers, 2004.

Piquemal, Michel, and Melissa Daly. *When Life Stinks: How to Deal with Your Bad Moods, Blues, and Depression.* New York, NY: Amulet Books, 2004.

Reber, Deborah. *Chill: Stress-Reducing Techniques for a More Balanced, Peaceful You.* New York, NY: Simon Pulse, 2008.

Russell, Craig. *Antidepressants and Side Effects.* Philadelphia, PA: Mason Crest Publishers, 2007.

Scowen, Kate. *My Kind of Sad: What It's Like to Be Young and Depressed.* New York, NY: Annick Press, 2006.

Walker, Maryalice. *The Development of Antidepressants: The Chemistry of Depression.* Philadelphia, PA: Mason Crest Publishers, 2007.

Zucker, Faye, and Joan E. Huebl. *Beating Depression: Teens Find Light at the End of the Tunnel.* New York, NY: Franklin Watts, 2007.

Index

About the Author

Judy Monroe Peterson has earned two master's degrees, including one in public health education, and is the author of more than fifty educational books for young people. She is a former health care, technical, and academic librarian and college faculty member; a biologist and research scientist; and curriculum editor with more than twenty-five years of experience. She has taught courses at 3M, the University of Minnesota, and Lake Superior College. Currently, she is a writer and editor of K–12 and post–high school curriculum materials on a variety of subjects, including health, life skills, biology, life science, and the environment.

Photo Credits